1

Thank you for purchasing this book

You may view Cariporter's website to learn more.

www.cariporter.ca

Don't Just Survive
The Crisis,

Become Healthy
And Wealthy Too

Learn to improve your health and finances

See how John Templeton and Warren Buffett

became wealthy from crisis

Make use of the opportunities during this

problem

LEROY A. BROWN

Cariporter Inc

Toronto

By reading this document, the reader agrees that under no circumstances is the author responsible for any losses, direct or indirect, which are incurred as a result of the use of information contained within this document, including, but not limited to, — errors, omissions, or inaccuracies.

For information about permission to reproduce selections from this book, write to info@cariporter.ca   or to Cariporter Inc, 465 Yonge St. P.O. Box 73021, Toronto, Ontario, M4Y 2W5, Canada.

www.cariporter.ca

ISBN 978-0-9936618-7-7 (paperback)
ISBN 978-0-9936618-8-4 (e-book)

TABLE OF CONTENTS

THANK YOU

Thank you, Paula and Jada, for your overall support.

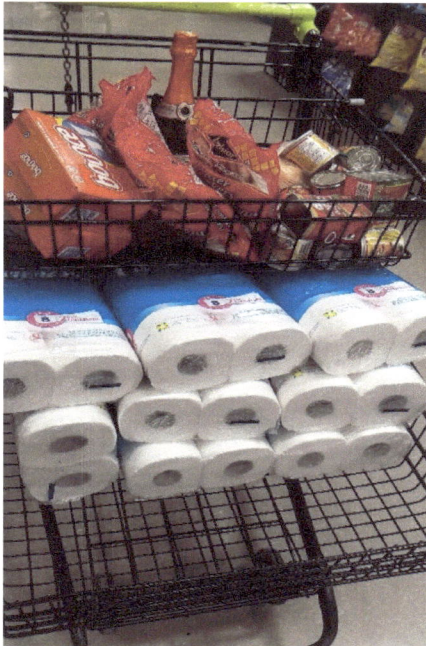

Toilet paper and some groceries were in high demand, causing scarcity during the coronavirus COVID-19 pandemic.

INTRODUCTION

Being able to manage your money is one of the most critical skills to possess in this day and age. Due to the ongoing changes in the world almost every day, being able to assess your financial situation is becoming increasingly important.

Keeping track of your finances is something you will want to be doing more often, especially if you're independent, or are new to the world of finances.

Knowing how to manage your money, how to save it, and where to invest it, is essential if you want to maintain financial security in life. Budgeting, banking, mortgages, insurance, investments, retirement planning, and tax management all sound like high-end terms, but are all terms that you will eventually need to understand if you wish to make sound financial decisions in life.

Nevertheless, being able to keep track of your finances does not necessarily have to be as daunting as it seems. I am here to help you in better understanding your financial situation, how you can make it better, and finally, start achieving your dreams.

Let's face it, everybody wants money, and there is almost no dream that does not require at least a small amount of money.

Therefore, being able to attract and manage money will help you get to your dreams faster. Whether you are a student, a new graduate, an employee for over thirty (30) years, or you have already retired, financial guidance is something everyone can make use of now.

Due to the current novel coronavirus COVID-19 pandemic, many economies across the globe have shut down, and we are likely heading into a predicted recession.

The novel coronavirus COVID-19, which is now officially called severe acute respiratory syndrome coronavirus 2 (SARS-COV-2), as its transmission becomes more expansive, has prompted healthcare experts to come up with better ways of stopping the spread. SARS-COV-2 is officially a pandemic, and getting back to your regular life may take longer than the next few weeks.

The pandemic might look like all gloom and doom, but it is the time to take stock of your finances and overall life. **It is time to reflect on your financial, mental, spiritual, emotional, psychological, and physical well-being.**

It is expected that an economic recession will happen soon, and that this future industrial decline will be worse than ever before.

With so many individuals and countries in debt, the recession will be a terrible time for everyone.

As countries continue to print more money to help prop up their economies, it is worsening the financial and overall economic outcomes.

Thus, it is with this and more in mind that I have decided to share valuable information with you.

I intend to help you manage and improve your finances, show you how others have gotten rich from crises, and help to guide you as to some of the things that you may do during this pandemic.

Do enjoy its contents, and may it be of great assistance to you in achieving your goals.

CHAPTER ONE - ASSESS YOUR FINANCIAL SITUATION

When it comes to personal finances, it may seem a bit difficult or overwhelming to find out where you are financially.

Nevertheless, it is essential to know where you stand in terms of money, so you may make any necessary adjustments to move forward.

Below are a few simple steps to help you in determining what your current financial situation is:

1. HAVE YOUR DOCUMENTS AT HAND

Having most (if not all) your documents present will be the first step to assessing your financial situation. You can do this online if you use the various accounting, bookkeeping, or budgeting tools that are available.

You may do like me and gather all your documents in paper format.

These documents can be mortgage agreement and payments, statements like bank account and credit card, and receipts for rent and property taxes.

2. CALCULATE YOUR NET WORTH

Net worth may sound like a big word, but it is merely the difference between your existing assets (things that give you money), and any liabilities (things that take money from you).

In this step, you will have to make two lists, one labeled assets, and the other liabilities.

Examples of **assets** are;

- House if it gives you money like rent
- Car if you rent it

- Money in bank account

- Stocks

- Land that you have rented to a farmer

- Lawnmower that you have rented

- Trademark that you have licensed to others to use

- Song you have produced and is earning royalties

- Book you have published and is earning income

- Website that you are earning from like selling advertising space

- Retirement savings like your RRSP (Registered Retirement Savings Plan) in Canada, and 401K Retirement Plan In The United States of America (U.S.A.)

Examples of **liabilities** are;

- House if you are not making money from it but you are paying the mortgage, or you are renting it, but the rent does not cover the expenses like your mortgage and repairs

- Car if you are not making money from it, but you're paying back the loan or maintaining it

- Stocks if they have lost value, e.g., you bought them for $100, and it has declined to $70

- Debt you owe on your credit card

- Tax returns fee if you pay someone to do it for you

- Insurance for your car, house, etc.
- Legal fees if you have to use a lawyer or paralegal for anything

- Utilities such as electricity and water

- Telephone bill

- Cable bill

- Streaming services bills such as Netflix and Amazon Prime

- Courses that you are doing and have to pay for

- Fee to renew road license for your vehicle

- Food you buy

- Coffee you may buy in the mornings

- Gas you purchase for your vehicle

- Vehicle repairs

- House repairs

- Landscaper for cutting your grass or any other services

- Student loan

After you have added up all your assets and then your liabilities, subtract the total liabilities from the total assets. The result after the subtraction is your net worth.

E.g.

Assets:

House	$750,000
Car	$25,000
Stocks	$15,000
Savings	$5,000
TOTAL	$795,000

Liabilities:

Mortgage owing	$350,000
House insurance	$5,000
Car insurance	$2,500
Credit card	$8,000
Student Loan	$35,000
TOTAL	$400,500

Assets	**$795,000**
Less Liabilities	**$400,500**
NET WORTH	**$394,500**

A positive net worth such as the example above is good because it means you can cover your expenses.

A negative net worth means you are not able to cover your expenses.

3. POSITIVE AND NEGATIVE NET WORTH

POSITIVE NET WORTH

A positive net worth such as the example above is good because it means you can cover your expenses.

This is where you want to be at all times. Not because it is less stressful, but you are better able to weather any financial challenges that will come your way, such as the expected recession.

Also, having positive net worth will help you to take advantage of opportunities that may present themselves.

For example, with the rental income and equity from the house you have rented you may get another loan to purchase another house for rent.

This other house you have bought and rented, will increase your assets and provide more income.

NEGATIVE NET WORTH

A negative net worth means you are **not** able to cover your expenses.

This is a position you want to avoid. This is because it makes it more challenging for you to deal with unpleasant circumstances such as becoming ill or weathering the expected recession.

4. HOW TO CHANGE NEGATIVE NET WORTH TO POSITIVE NET WORTH

There are two (2) ways to change negative net worth to positive net worth.

1.

Reduce your liabilities, so it is less than your assets.

For example, if you shop around, you may find cheaper insurance for your car. Do ensure you are ok with the coverage you are getting.

Another example is, pay more than the minimum payment on your credit card debt so that you are reducing the principal and interest at the same time faster.

2.

Increasing your assets so it is more than your liabilities.

For example, you may purchase a stock for $25, and it goes up to $135. Now, if you had bought one hundred (100) of these stocks for $2,500, then you now have $13,500.

Another example is, you may start renting the upper part of your house, and you stay in the basement. This rent may be enough to cover expenses and your mortgage.

5. SOME CALCULATIONS THAT MAY BE OF IMPORTANCE TO YOU

Please note the following:

1. You may see in other sources that the ratios may be called different names.

For example, **credit – market debt to disposable income ratio** is the same as **debt to disposable income ratio**

2. Calculations may be slightly different from other sources

3. In the calculations, you may multiply the ratio by 100 to get the percentage.

For example, the debt to disposable income ratio may be determined as follows:

A. Debt

Mortgage owing	$250,000
Line of credit	$20,000
Student loan	$32,000
TOTAL	$302,000

B. Disposable Income

Money earned as Operations Manager	$120,000
Less 33% income tax	$39,600
TOTAL	$80,400

C. <u>Debt to Disposable Income Ratio</u>

Debt to disposable income ratio = <u>debt/</u>

Disposable income

Debt to disposable income ratio = <u>$302,000/</u>   = 3.756

$80,400

Percentage is 3.756 x 100 = 375.6%

<u>3.756 Ratio means</u>

The 3.756 ratio means you will need at least 3.756 (almost 4) times your after-tax income to pay off your debt.

<u>375.6% Percentage means</u>

The 375.6% means your debt is 375.6 % (almost 400%) of your after-tax income.

LIQUIDITY RATIO

Liquidity is your ability to trade your assets for cash.

Monetary assets are the easiest to change into cash.

Examples of monetary assets are cash in your bank account, money market funds, saving bonds, and cash in the safe in your house.

It is suggested that monetary assets should be able to cover your monthly liabilities such as electricity bills, groceries, insurance, etc. for at least six (6) months.

It is calculated as:

Liquidity ratio = monetary assets/
Monthly expenses

EMERGENCY FUND RATIO

This is mostly having cash that can help to cover your expenses for several months when unforeseen events happen, such as job loss, death in the family, and the current coronavirus COVID-19 pandemic.

It is calculated as:

Emergency ratio = no. of months x total monthly
expenses

TARGETED NET WORTH RATIO

This gives you an indication of what you should be worth concerning your income and age.

It is calculated as:

Targeted Net Worth Ratio = age x (pretax income)/
10

CURRENT RATIO

The current ratio simply test if you can pay back short term liabilities such as a 30-day loan and property taxes, using your short term assets (liquid assets), such as money in your savings account, and government bonds.

A ratio of 1 or higher means you have more short term assets than debts which is an excellent position to be.

It is calculated as:

Current Ratio = short term cash assets/
short term liabilities

DEBT-TO-ASSET RATIO

The ratio tells how much debt you have compared to your assets.

The higher the ratio, such as 0.50 and above, the worse your situation.

The lower the ratio such as 0.10 and below, the better your position.

This ratio involves your assets such as the house you are renting, and the cash in your high-interest savings account (HISA). It also includes your liabilities such as mortgage and student loans.

Total Debt-To-Asset Ratio = total liabilities/

total assets

DEBT-TO-INCOME RATIO

This ratio tells if your debt (liabilities like student and mortgage loans) is too high when compared to your income.

It is considered bad if the amount of money you owe (i.e. debt) is 0.30 or higher. It means you are using 30% of your income to pay your debt.

Debt-To-Income Ratio = annual debt repayments/

Gross   income

DEBT-TO-DISPOSABLE INCOME RATIO

Disposable income is the amount of money you have after paying taxes.

Debt may include mortgage liabilities, line of credit, and nonmortgage loans such as student and car loans.

So the debt-to-disposable income ratio shows if your debt is too much for the money you have left after taxes, or if you have enough disposable income to pay down debt, save, invest, pay bills, and buy household items such as groceries.

Debt-To- Disposable Income Ratio = debt/

Disposable Income

It is said that 0.14 or lower means you have sufficient disposable income, whereas 0.15 or higher may mean you have too much debt.

COST OF DEBT

The cost of debt indicates if your interest on a loan is going to be high or low, depending on how much debt you have.

This can also be determined by your credit score, where less than 650 will usually make your interest rate higher because lenders such as banks and credit unions, see you as a risky borrower.

If your credit score is higher than 650, then your interest rate will be lower.

For example:

1. You borrowed $200,000 from the credit union at 6% interest rate.

2. You also borrowed $100,000 from your friend at 4% interest rate.

3. The interest rate you will pay is:

(a) 6% x $200,000 = $12,000

(b) 4% x $100,000 = $4,000

(c) Total interest = $12,000 + $4,000 = $16,000

(d) Total debt = $200,000 + $100,000 = $300,000

The interest rate (cost of debt) you will pay is

$$\frac{\$16,000}{\$300,000} \times 100 = 5.3\%$$

SOLVENCY RATIO

The solvency ratio shows if you can pay off all your debt with the assets you have now.

Solvency Ratio $= \dfrac{\text{net worth}}{\text{total assets}}$

INVESTMENT ASSETS-TO-TOTAL ASSETS RATIO

This tells you how much of your assets you have put to use for profitable returns.

Investment assets are usually liquid assets such as stocks, bonds, and money market funds.

A ratio of 0.10 or 10% and higher is considered excellent.

Investment Assets-To-Total

Assets Ratio = <u>investment assets/</u>

total assets

6. BUDGET YOUR MONEY AND KEEP TRACK OF IT

Making a budget is great because you get to know how much you can spend. It also helps you to decide on what you are going to spend on and keep track of all purchases.

Now, remember what Robert Kiyosaki author of *Rich dad Poor Dad* keeps saying when you receive your income – "**PAY YOURSELF FIRST.**"

Some say you pay yourself at least ten percent (10%) of your income, and as your financial situation gets better, you may go up to even fifty percent (50%).

If your financial situation is horrible, you may want to pay yourself at five percent (5%) or even lower.

It doesn't matter what amount you pay yourself. The main thing is to ensure you are paying yourself first.

It has been suggested that the amount you pay yourself goes towards your savings, investments, and business (if you started one or planned to).

The rest of your income will go towards bills and expenses such as groceries.

For example:

1.

Your annual income	$45,000
Less 12% income tax	$5,400
Disposable income	$39,600

2. Pay yourself first 10%

    $39,600 x 10% = $3,960 per year

    $3,960 /   = $330 per month
    12

3. Remaining disposable income

    $39, 600 - $3,960 = $35,640 per year

    $35,640/   = $2,970 per month
    12

4. Spending budget for $3,960

RRSP $1,000

(Registered Retirement Savings Plan)

Buy stocks $1,000

Internet marketing $500

(For products you are selling online)

Emergency Fund	$1,000
High-Interest Savings Account	$460
TOTAL	$3,960

5. Spending budget for $35,640

Property tax	$1,200
Mortgage	$21,000
Groceries	$4,800
Credit card payments	$1,440
Gas for vehicle	$2,400
Insurance & license for vehicle	$1,540
Miscellaneous (e.g. donations, utilities, etc.)	$3,260
TOTAL	$35,640

7. MAKE FINANCIAL GOALS

Now that you know where you are financially, you now have to decide what it is that you want to do.

Do you want to earn more money and how much?

Do you want to pay off your debts within two (2) years?

Do you want to go on a vacation when this pandemic is over, and it is safe to do so?

Do you want to buy another house or a condo?

Are you going to move your parents in so you can take better care of them?

Do you want to start or increase your emergency fund?

Do you want to start or increase the education fund for your children?

Do you want to increase your retirement savings?

Do you want to improve and increase your investments?

These are just some of the questions you might ask yourself.

When you have decided which question it is, and what is the specific goal, then do what Napoleon Hill author of *Think and Grow Rich* said "**BEGIN IMMEDIATELY.**"

Begin immediately working and putting your plan into action. It doesn't matter if the procedure is complete, or you do not have all the resources needed, such as the amount of money it is going to take.

The most important thing here is getting started and being persistent until you have achieved your goal.

So these steps will help you to arrive at your goal:

1st Figure out what is your goal

This has already been explained above by asking questions.

2nd Create a plan

Part of this has been explained above. But we are going to go a bit further.

It is a good idea to ensure your plan is SMART i.e., specific, measurable, achievable, relevant, and timely.

Specific

This means your plan should be simple; you know exactly what you want, well thought out, and is of importance.

Measurable

This means you can track your progress to see if you are accomplishing your goal or not, and when you have reached that goal.

Achievable

This means that the goal you have can be accomplished.

Relevant

This means that your goal corresponds with your financial situation.

Time

Time simply means that the goal will be done by a certain date.

3rd Begin immediately

You must begin immediately to implement your plan and get closer to your goal. This is because you will start developing momentum, and eventually, you will become motivated and confident.

EXAMPLE

After finding out where you are financially, you have now decided that paying off your credit card principal and interest will be best for you at this time.

You also know this is a SMART goal because:

SPECIFIC

(a) WHAT

What are you trying to get done? This is the question you are answering. And the answer you have given is, "I want to pay off my credit card interest and principal."

(b) WHY

Why do you want to pay off your credit card interest and principal?

Your answer to this question is - paying off your credit card allows you to:

- Have more money to spend on other things
- Better handle any event in your life such as a job loss, because you can focus on finding a job, or starting a business without worrying about credit card payments
- Put the money that was going to credit card payments towards your retirement savings

- Improve your credit score

- Have better mental health as you don't have to be worried, or feel overwhelmed by the amount of credit card debt you have to pay

- Feel more confident as this burden of paying off your credit card principal and interest is no longer there

- Have better health as you are less stressed and your blood pressure is better controlled because you are not pressured to make payments on your credit card anymore

- Have a better marriage as you have fewer arguments about finances

- Have fewer bills to pay, which will make you feel better and even motivated

(c) WHO

Who is where you have identified that you are going to be the one to pay off your credit card balance.

(d) WHERE

You have selected the specific credit card you are going to pay off and the financial institution through which you are going to make the payments.

(e) WHICH

Which path am I going to take to pay off my credit card?

You have decided you are going to work overtime and use that extra money to pay off my credit card debt. You may also add, choose one, or make use of several of the following paths:

- Transfer the debt on my credit card to another credit card that has a lower interest rate.
- You may consolidate your credit card and other debts into a personal loan at a lower interest rate.
- You may call your credit card issuer and negotiate a lower interest rate.

- You may call your credit card issuer and negotiate a three (3) to six (6) months no interest period, so allowing you to pay down your debt faster.

- Make use of your credit card insurance (if you have one).

- Make use of government-approved debt counseling.

- Stop using your credit card while you continue to make the monthly payments.

- Each month you pay more than the minimum payment, so you are reducing the interest and principal at the same time faster.

MEASURABLE

To be able to know if you are getting closer to achieving your goal, you may compare your current credit card statement with the previous one each month. If you see that the balance is getting less each month, it means you are progressing towards your goal of paying off your credit card debt.

ACHIEVABLE

You know you can pay off your credit card because you are currently making payments, and you are determined to accomplish this goal.

RELEVANT

You realize that this is important because it is part of your efforts to be in a better financial position.

TIME

Based on the number of monthly payments you will have to make, you now know it will take you eighteen (18) months or one and a half (1 ½) year to pay off your credit card debt.

Therefore, by October 31, 2021, you will pay off your credit card debt.

CHAPTER TWO – HOW THEY GOT RICH FROM A CRISIS

HOW JOHN TEMPLETON BECAME RICH DURING THE 1929 – 1939 GREAT DEPRESSION AND WORLD WAR II 1939 - 1945

Sir John Templeton was born in 1912 in Winchester, Tennessee, in The United States of America (U.S.A.). He attended Yale and Oxford Universities.

1929 STOCK MARKET CRASH

By the 1920s, investors were very optimistic about the stock market, especially when they heard of regular people like bus drivers, teachers, etc. becoming millionaires from investing in it.

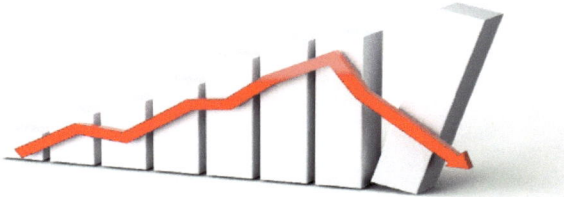

Image by Mediamodifier from Pixabay

Individuals, banks, and other investors were so convinced that they even borrowed money to invest in the stock market.

In early 1929, the stock market had declined but was propped up by the banks that restored confidence.

Commerce such as steel production and car sales had slowed, banks were closing as they weren't able to resolve their cash flow problems. But the stock market was still vibrant thanks to its positive investors.

In early October 1929, the British Finance Minister was pessimistic about the U.S. stock market. Then major media outlets like The Wall Street Journal, New York Times and the Associated Press began reporting negative news about the U.S. stock market.

Later in October 1929, the economist Irving Fisher wrote in the New York Times newspaper that the U.S. stock market prices were at their highest.

On October 24, 1929, the stock market began its four - day crash.

Some of the highlights of the four-day crash are:

- City Services utility holding company made the biggest bloc trade of over 140,000 shares.
- Montgomery-Ward and other big names declined in market value.
- There was mass panic that led to mass selling, especially when money borrowed to buy stocks

could not be repaid immediately, and margin calls were made.

The 1929 stock market crash saw the fall in stock prices, and the Dow Jones Industrial Average dropped over 20%. This made it one of the worse declines in U.S. history.

Because of the overconfidence in the stock market that fueled its exponential growth, individuals, and other investors were hard hit as the prices came tumbling down.

The stock market decline led to individuals and families losing their life savings, among other negative outcomes. This contributed to the Great Depression that followed.

1929 – 1939 THE GREAT DEPRESSION

The Great Depression started at different times in countries around the world. But it can be said to have started in 1929 in the U.S., as there was already a decline in economic production, increase in unemployment, high amounts of debt, etc.

The U.S. stock market collapse in October 1929 simply accelerated The Great Depression and made it worse.

HOW JOHN TEMPLETON BECAME RICH

After the stock market crash in 1929 and the U.S. began to recover from The Great Depression in 1939, Hitler led Germany to invade Poland. This prompted England and France to declare war against Germany in retaliation.

This 1939 invasion by Germany essentially started World War II, which was from 1939-1945.

The 1939 invasion caused great pessimism in countries like Canada and the United States of America (U.S.A.).

This despair caused falls in stock prices.

It was this decline in stock prices that John Templeton saw an opportunity.

To take advantage of the drop in share prices in the U.S., John Templeton borrowed US$10,000 (about US$185,000 in 2020) to purchase one hundred (100) shares in as many New York Stock Exchange-listed companies as possible, that were selling for $1 a share or less.

He eventually invested in a total of one hundred and four (104) companies, of which, thirty-four (34) were in bankruptcy.

Four (4) years later, he sold the stocks he bought and made about US$40,000 (about US$573,000 in 2020). This is approximately four hundred percent (400%) return on his investment.

In 1954, John Templeton entered the mutual fund market by creating the Templeton Growth Fund.

He was also the first in the United States of America (U.S.A.) to start a mutual fund that invests globally.

By 1959, John Templeton had created five (5) funds with over US$66 million under management. That same year he took his funds public.

Going public simply means, he offered stocks to anyone and entities so they can own equity in the company.

He used his mutual funds to invest in Japan in the 1960s and 1970s.

He started investing globally after traveling to different countries and realizing the opportunities that they presented.

In 1964, John Templeton renounced his U.S. citizenship to avoid income tax payments, and lived in Nassau, Bahamas as a British citizen.

By 1992, John Templeton's company was called Templeton, Galbraith & Hansberger and had over seventy (70) mutual funds worldwide with over $20 billion under management.

His company was located in Nassau, Bahamas.

It was in 1992 that 79 years old John Templeton decided to merge his company with Franklin Resources, to ensure the continued stability of his clients' investments.

This merger created the largest public mutual fund company in the U.S.

John Templeton was well recognized as a value investor and died in 2008 in Nassau, Bahamas where he lived for most of his remaining life.

HOW WARREN BUFFETT PROFITED FROM THE 2008 SUBPRIME & FINANCIAL CRISES

Warren Buffett was born in 1930 in Omaha, Nebraska in The United States of America (U.S.A.). He attended the Wharton School of the University of Pennsylvania, University of Nebraska, Columbia Business School, and New York Institute of Finance.

2007 – 2010 SUBPRIME MORTGAGE CRISIS

The U.S. subprime mortgage crisis was a financial disaster across the United States of America (U.S.A.),

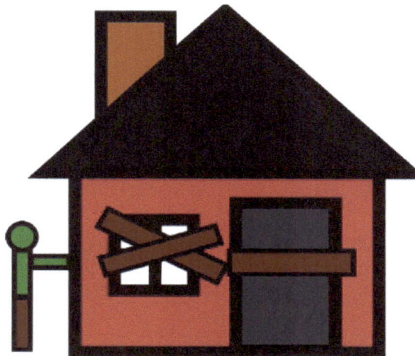

Image by Clker-Free-Vector-Images from Pixabay

that contributed to the U.S. recession that was from 2007 – 2009.

One of the things that caused the subprime mortgage crisis was the decline in house value, which helped to cause mortgage delinquencies, foreclosures, and reduction in mortgage- backed securities.

Mortgage delinquency is the nonpayment of a loan that is secured by real estate or property.

Foreclosures in this crisis were the sale of houses that were used as collateral for loans such as mortgages. The houses were sold to recover the remaining amount that wasn't paid.

Mortgage-backed securities are investments that are made up of house loans (mortgages) that are bought from the bank that issued them.

Subprime lending is simply the giving of loans to individuals who may not be able to repay.

2007 – 2009 FINANCIAL CRISIS

The subprime market crash eventually led to a financial crisis in the United States of America (U.S.A.). This

financial crisis expanded into the global financial crisis (GFC).

Some highlights of the financial crisis are:

- Lehman Brothers, a global financial firm and one of the largest investment banks collapsed in 2008 after the Federal Reserve decided not to guarantee its loans.

- New Century Financial Corporation, a real estate investment trust, had to file for bankruptcy as it could not fulfill its financial obligations.

- Federal rates were eventually reduced to 0%.

- The Federal Reserve started to give short-term credit to banks with subprime mortgages.

- Bear Stearns, a global investment firm, brokerage, and securities trader was one of the largest investment banks in the U.S., saw a big decline in its market value, because of information being circulated that customers were withdrawing their money.

  Eventually, Bear Stearns had its bad loans guaranteed by the Federal Reserves. This enabled it to be purchased by JPMorgan Chase in 2008.

- IndyMac, one of the largest savings and loans association and mortgage providers in the United States of America (U.S.A.) failed in 2008.

Part of its failure was because its mortgage operations were negatively affected by the subprime mortgage crisis.

- The Dow Jones Industrial Average, a stock market index that measures the performance of about 30 large companies listed on the stock exchanges in the United States of America (U.S.A.), dropped to over seven hundred (700) points in 2008.

- Washington Mutual, one of the largest savings and loan association in the U.S., went bankrupt after many customers went to withdraw their money, and they were also negatively affected by mortgage defaults.

- The Big Three automobile manufacturers (i.e., General Motors, Ford, and Fiat Chrysler (FCA US)) were bailed out.

- Many debtors could not make their regular mortgage payments.

HOW WARREN BUFFETT BECAME WEALTHIER

In 1956, Warren Buffett started Buffett Associates Limited and created more partnerships as he uses the funds from these agreements to invest in companies.

In 1962, he merged all these arrangements into one business called Buffett Partnerships Limited.

In the same year, Warren Buffet began buying shares in Berkshire Hathaway, a textile manufacturing company.

By 1963, Buffett became the largest shareholder of Berkshire Hathaway and eventually became its Chairman and Chief Executive Officer (CEO).

In 2008, while many were going bankrupt, and there was great pessimism during the subprime mortgage and financial crises, Warren Buffett, saw several opportunities and acted on them.

There were several investments Warren Buffett made, and of these, we have selected the following:

- In 2008 around April, Warren Buffett helped the popular candy maker Mars to finance the US$23 billion purchase of Wrigley.

  The arrangement saw Warren Buffett lending Mars about US$4.4 billion and taking a minority stake (about 10%) in Wrigley for US$2.1 billion.

  By 2016, it was reported that Warren Buffett made at least US$680 million on his investment.

- In September 2008, Goldman Sachs announced that it would receive funding from Warren Buffett as part of its efforts to raise capital during the financial crisis.

Warren Buffett invested in Goldman Sachs by purchasing preferred stocks for approximately US$5 billion.

In 2011, Goldman Sachs bought back the preferred shares from Warren Buffett giving him about US$500 million in bonus.

- In October 2008, Warren Buffett provided about US$3 billion to General Electric (GE), which was aiming to raise US$12 billion to beef up its finances to help survive the crisis.

The deal involved purchasing preferred shares at a ten percent (10%) dividend. Also, Buffett was offered to buy common stocks at a discount.

By 2017, Warren Buffett had recovered his investment making at least US$300 million in profits.

CHAPTER THREE – THE CURRENT CRISIS-CORONAVIRUS COVID-19 SEVERE ACUTE RESPIRATORY SYNDROME CORONAVIRUS 2 (SARS-COV-2) PANDEMIC

The current crisis affecting the world now is the novel coronavirus COVID-19 or severe acute respiratory syndrome coronavirus 2 (SARS-COV-2) pandemic.

SARS-COV-2 is a newly discovered virus that affects your respiratory system. It can be mild as well as severe to the point of death.

This virus is believed by many to be deliberately created to spread globally.

Many individuals are even skeptical about the vaccines companies and countries are hurrying to produce.

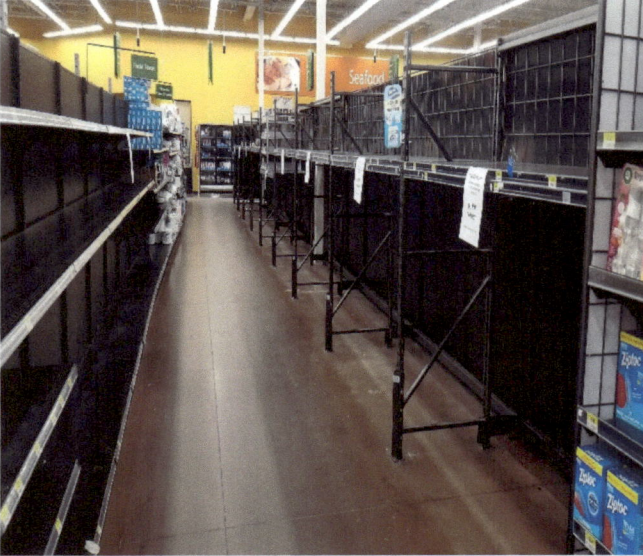

Empty shelves in grocery store during the coronavirus COVID-19 pandemic

The worldwide spread of this virus has caused many countries to close their borders, shut down businesses, close schools, and require all its citizens to stay inside.

Some countries have even declared a state of emergency.

Symptoms

Signs that you or others might have this virus are:

- Coughing (usually a dry cough)
- Having fever
- Having difficulty breathing
- Developing pneumonia after a while

While some individuals have reported not developing symptoms, most do within fourteen (14) days.

Prevention

The three (3) best ways to protect yourself from being infected from this virus are:

1. Wash your hands
2. Stay away from others
3. Maintain or boost your immune system

CANADA

According to the Ontario.ca website, by April 24, 2020 at 10.30 am in Ontario – the largest and most populated province in Canada, there were 13,519 reported cases of people being infected with this disease. Of this number, 7,087 were resolved, 763 died, 910 were hospitalized, 243 were in Intensive Care Unit (ICU), and 193 were on ventilators in the ICU.

According to the website Canada.ca, by April 24, 2020, there were 42,750 reported cases and 2,197 deaths.

UNITED STATES OF AMERICA (U.S.A.)

According to the washingtonpost.com website, over 870,000 persons have been infected with the virus. Of this number, over 50,000 have died, and almost half (1/2) of this happened in New York.

GLOBALLY

According to the worldometers.info website, over 2.8 million persons have been infected with the virus. Of this number, over 195,000 have died.

HAPPENINGS

MEDICAL

- You may take the self-assessment test to know if you might have the coronavirus at https://covid-19.ontario.ca/self-assessment/.

- The United Kingdom (U.K.) Prime Minister Boris Johnson, his Health Secretary Matt Hancock, and Chris Whitty – Chief Medical Officer tested positive or had the symptoms of the coronavirus.

  U.K. Prime Minister Boris Johnson was eventually treated in the intensive care unit (ICU) and survived.

- President Andry Rajoelina of Madagascar, have announced that his country has developed a herbal product called COVID-Organics, which can help to cure individuals from the coronavirus.

  It had its first COVID-19 case by March 28, 2020.

- Smithfield Foods Inc. is a global food company, the world's largest pork processor, hog producer, and headquartered in Smithfield, Virginia, in the United States (U.S.).

  It has confirmed a specific case of one of its employees having the coronavirus by March 28, 2020.

SOCIAL

- The MS Zaandam cruise ship owned by Holland America had four (4) of its passengers died on board.

  This ship which was touring South America before the World Health Organization (WHO) declared the coronavirus a pandemic on March 11, 2020, was left stranded at sea as countries closed their ports.

  Its fellow ship – MS Rotterdam came to rescue it with medical personnel, supplies, etc.

  MS Zaandam was eventually allowed to dock in Fort Everglades in Florida, United States (U.S.).

- Charities in Toronto distributed tents to homeless people because they thought it was better for the homeless individuals to camp outside in the ravines than in the city's overcrowded shelters, where they might be more susceptible to catching the coronavirus.

- Shrey Jain is an engineering science student at the University of Toronto who created a crowdsourcing website with his peers.

  The website is called flatten.ca, and it basically asks people to report symptoms or lack of them anonymously. This data is then mapped by postal code to create a coronavirus data outline.

- Frontline workers such as doctors, nurses, police officers, firefighters, etc. may send their children to emergency child care in Canada.

- American pop singer Lady Gaga, raised over US$120 million from her One World: Together at Home benefit concern on April 18, 2020 for health care workers.

ECONOMIC

- By March 28, 2020

    - Apple, Microsoft, Amazon, Facebook, and Google had their market value declined by an estimated total of US$1 trillion.

    - For over two (2) weeks, Apple and Android saw app sales growth of about US$1 billion.

    - Amazon advertised that it would be hiring 100,000 workers to meet demand.

    - Since the coronavirus pandemic started, there was approximately sixty-six percent (66%) increase in the number of Netflix app downloaded in Italy.

    - It was stated that Microsoft saw a thirty-seven percent (37%) rise in the use of its Microsoft teams messaging and collaboration tools.

- Canada and other countries like the United States (U.S.), and Germany printed over US$5 trillion in debt to be used as relief packages.

- According to a report by the consultancy firm Bain, the luxury goods market is expected to shrink by about 15% – 35%.

- Luxury retailers such as the United Kingdom's Burberry Group PLC have announced that sales could fall by as much as fifty percent (50%).

Kering has also announced that sales are expected to decline by fifteen percent (15%).

Some of the brands owned by Kering are Gucci, Bottega Veneta, Saint Laurent, Alexander McQueen, Balenciaga, Brioni, Christopher Kane, McQ, Volcom, Cobra, Stella Mccartney, and Tomas   Maier.

- As commercial flights decrease, private flights have increased.

One company that has decided to take advantage of the demand is VistaJet.

VistaJet is a global aircraft services provider that has acted upon the demand by offering short-term leases for charter-plane customers, where they may have exclusive access to private aircraft for them to travel.

VistaJet is headquartered in Malta.

- According to the Canadian newspaper York Region Review April 2020, over eighty percent (>80%) of service-based workers were negatively impacted by the closure of restaurants, shops, hotels, etc.

It was also stated that only a small number of these individuals had employment insurance (EI).

- Walmart Canada plans to hire ten thousand (10,000) individuals.

- Walmart, Loblaws, and other grocery retailers in Canada have increased hourly wages by CAD$2 per hour as danger pay or premium.

- Walmart Canada has given its employees a one-time bonus of up to CAD$200, for their dedication and hard work during the current pandemic.

- Medical doctors, nurses, etc., and related entities are declared critical services in Canada, and as such, are allowed to be open.

- Grocery stores, auto shops, etc., and related entities are recognized as essential services in Canada, and as such, are allowed to be open.

- Companies like Cargill, Maple Leaf Foods Inc., Campbell Soup Company, Mondelez International Inc., Kraft Heinz Company, and Hormel Foods Corporation are paying bonuses or premiums to their workers.

- Dairy producers in Vermont, United States (U.S.) are sending request to volunteers to help milk cows if farmers fall ill.

- Many realtors are using Facebook Live for open houses.

- This was happening before the pandemic and is continuing, as Saudi Arabia produces more oil in its price war with Russia. This has led to a significant drop in gas prices.

For example, in the Greater Toronto Area (GTA) in Ontario, Canada, gas prices have fallen from as high as CAD$1.60 to as low as CAD$0.64.

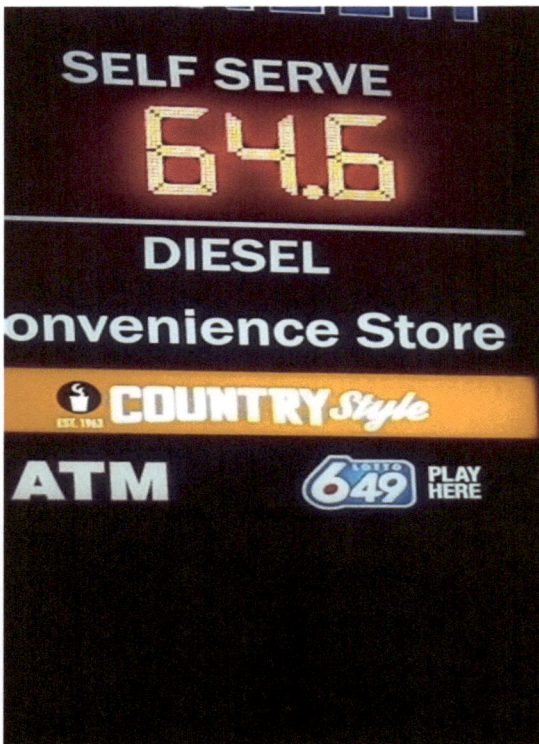

Low gas price in Markham, Ontario, Canada

- Because of the price war between Saudi Arabia and Russia, the pandemic, and other factors, Enerplus Corporation saw its stock price declining by about thirty-seven percent (37%) on Monday, March 9, 2020.

  Cenovus Energy Inc. saw its share price fall by approximately fifty-two (52%) for similar reasons as Enerplus Corp.

- International freight and logistics companies are reporting as much as eighty-five percent (85%) decline in the volume of Chinese-made goods.

- According to the Canadian newspaper Financial Post March 11, 2020, Canada has always had a driver shortage, and it appears to be getting worse.

  It has been estimated that there are over 20,000 job   vacancies.

- On Monday, March 9, 2020 the S&P/TSX Composite Index declined by just over ten percent (10%) and was considered the most significant one-day drop since October 19, 1987.

The S&P/TSX Composite Index is the Canadian benchmark index. It represents most of the major Canadian companies on the stock exchange.

The S&P/TSX Composite Index mainly shows how the major companies are performing.

The S&P means Standard and Poors, and TSX means the Toronto Stock Exchange.

The TSX is Canada's primary stock market and is considered the ninth (9th) largest in the world, according to the total market capitalization of its listed companies.

The S&P is a financial services provider in the U.S. It provides services such as credit ratings and financial market intelligence.

- By March 11, 2020, Tilray saw its market value falling by about sixty percent (60%).

  Tilray is a global Canadian company incorporated in the U.S., and trades on the NASDAQ stock exchange.

  Tilray does cannabis research, processing, harvesting, and distributing.

  Other cannabis companies such as Canopy Growth Corporation and Aurora Cannabis Inc. experienced declines as well.

- By March 11, 2020, Italy had announced plans to have a large scale moratorium on debt repayments, such as mortgages for families and businesses.

- Warren Buffett's Geico company is offering US$2.5 billion in credits to its approximately 19 million auto and motorcycle policyholders because the pandemic has reduced driving and riding.

  Allstate has also offered to return over US$600 million to its approximately 18 million policyholders.

CHAPTER FOUR – OPPORTUNITIES THAT EXIST IN THIS CURRENT CRISIS

Just like the good fortunes that existed during the 1929 – 1939 Great Depression, and the 2007 – 2009 financial crisis, such good events are happening during the current pandemic.

Some can make you extremely rich, while some will allow you to get through this pandemic in a financially stable way.

There are also health benefits to be gained from this health crisis.

Some of these opportunities are:

MONEY

FINANCIAL ASSISTANCE

This is where you can use various financial assistance being made available, to help you keep your financial situation and business stable.

CANADA

- Financial help from the Government of Canada

From the website https://www.canada.ca/en/department-finance/economic-response-plan.html you may learn more about the following financial assistance programs and others:

INDIVIDUALS

1. The Canadian government, together with the provinces and territories, will provide additional money to low income (earning less than CAD$2,500 per month on a full-time basis) essential workers.

2. The Canadian government will provide an extra CAD$300 per child through the Canada Child Benefit (CCB).

3. The Canadian government will provide a one-time special payment through the Goods and Services Tax Credit for low and modest-income families.

4. For individuals who have a loss of income, they may receive CAD$2,000 every four (4) weeks for up to sixteen (16) weeks.

5. The Canadian government is providing CAD$350 million to the Indigenous Community Support Fund, to address immediate needs in First Nations, Inuit, and Metis Nation communities.

6. Canadian banks are working with their customers, to help them with their mortgages, such as deferring their payments for up to six (6) months.

BUSINESSES

1. Through the Canada Emergency Wage Subsidy (CEWS), the Canadian government will be providing wage subsidies of up to seventy-five percent (75%).

2. The Canadian government has decided to allow employers to reduce the amount of payroll deduction remitted to the Canada Revenue

Agency (CRA) through the Temporary 10% Wage Subsidy.

3. The Canadian government is extending the Work-Sharing program for employers. This is to help provide income support to employees eligible for Employment Insurance (EI).

4. The Canadian government is providing additional loan support through the Business Development Bank of Canada (BDC), and Export Development Canada (EDC), via its Business Credit Availability Program (BCAP).

5. The Canadian government is providing interest - free loans of up to $40,000 to small businesses through the Canada Emergency Business Account (CEBA).

6. The Canadian federal government will provide up to CAD$306.8 million to help small and medium-sized indigenous businesses.

This will be done through Aboriginal Financial Institutions and will be administered by the National Aboriginal Capital Corporations Association, the Metis Capital Corporations, and Indigenous Services Canada.

7. The Canadian government will purchase up to CAD$150 billion of insured mortgage pools to help stabilize banks and mortgage lenders.

This will be done through the Canada Mortgage and Housing Corporation (CMHC) via the Insured Mortgage Purchase Program.

UNITED STATES OF AMERICA (USA)

You may go to the website

https://www.benefits.gov/help/faq/Coronavirus-resources to learn more about the benefits the U.S. government and states have for individuals and businesses.

INTERNATIONAL

You may go to the website

https://www.imf.org/en/About/FAQ/imf-response-to-covid-19#Q1 to learn more about what the International Monetary Fund (IMF) is doing to help the countries in its program.

JOBS

If there was ever a time you wanted a job, or just to earn extra money, now is that time.

Several jobs are in high demand, and the compensation for some are much better than before.

Some may just be for the pandemic period, while some may become permanent.

Some of these jobs may even be a step down for you, or maybe a step up depending on how you look at it.

Here are some job opportunities you may consider:

- Amazon wants to hire one hundred thousand (100,000) individuals, so whether you are in Canada, the U.S., etc. go ahead, get the information and apply.

- Walmart has always been hiring, and even more now. In Canada alone, it wants to hire more than ten thousand (10,000) persons.

- The Ontario provincial government in Canada has developed a website for anyone to find a job in the agriculture, agri-food, and food industry. You may visit the website https://www.ontario.ca/page/agriculture-and-food-jobs-ontario to learn more.

- The government of Canada also has the Youth Employment and Skills Strategy Program (https://www.canada.ca/en/employment-social-development/services/funding/youth-employment-skills-strategy-program.html), in which young individuals can participate.

  It is being expanded in order to create about one hundred and sixteen thousand (116,000) jobs, placements, and training opportunities.

- You may do food delivery, as many establishments are doing take-outs. So you may want to check out Uber Eats, Doordash, Skip the Dishes, etc.

- There are grocery stores that have seen great increases in purchases on their websites, as individuals choose to have groceries delivered to them, or do curbside pickups.

  So go ahead and get the information from your grocery stores in your town or city. You may also view sites like Walmart, Instacart, Costco, Grocery Gateway, etc.

- As persons do their best to avoid crowds, you may want to participate in the drive economy. You may visit sites like Uride, Uber, etc.

- Truck drivers have always been in demand, and now is no different. So check out sites like Indeed, ZipRecruiter, TruckerSearch.com, etc.

- You may help in the direct fight again the coronavirus by being a cleaner for infection control cleaning.

- As teleconferencing, telecommunication, cloud, and information technology (IT) services increase, more individuals are needed to maintain these services. So go ahead check out various IT jobs, sites like Microsoft Team, Zoom, Blackberry, Bell, Oracle, etc.

- Telehealth service providers like Babylon Health are hiring.

- You may use FlexJobs, Indeed, ZipRecruiter, etc. to find online jobs.

- You may do virtual babysitting through sites like Weneeddatenight.com, Sittercity, etc.

ONLINE & OFFLINE BUSINESSES

With more people using the internet now, the possibilities of earning an income online have become more positive.

Here are some of these good fortunes you may consider:

- With health being of the highest priority and even more so now, this is a great time to participate in the health sector.

  Some ways to do so are:

  1. Sell health products online without ever having to handle the products yourself. You may visit the website https://cariporterinc.puretrimgo.com/ to learn more.

Please note Cariporter Inc. is associated with this entity.

2. Make and sell masks online.

3. Make and sell sanitizers online.

4. You may supply needed health-related products to the government of Canada. You may visit https://buyandsell.gc.ca/calling-all-suppliers-help-canada-combat-covid-19 to learn more.

- As many kids are home, you may tutor online. So visit sites like Chegg Tutors, First Tutors, Outschool, etc. or start your own.

- You may offer your skills through sites such as Fiverr, Guru, and so on.

INVESTMENTS

STOCK MARKET

When the severe acute respiratory syndrome coronavirus 2 (SARS-COV-2) was declared a pandemic between March 11, 2020, and the next morning, stock prices eventually fell. Had investments been made then, you would have seen a price increase by now. And if you exercised your shares, such as selling them, you would have received your profit.

That doesn't mean that these good fortunes do not exist now; they are still there. You just have to do your research and then make your investment.

Currently, many stock market analysts are discussing if the lowest prices of stocks have been reached, so as to buy them as cheap as possible. But it appears no one knows for sure.

Nevertheless, do your research and make your investment.

Below I will show you real examples of stocks that did well, some of which you might already know.

Please note that stock prices are closing prices that have been adjusted for dividends and splits.

- Netflix

Netflix Inc. is a media services provider and production company located in Los Gatos, California, U.S.A.

Its stock symbol is NFLX, and it trades on the NASDAQ.

Because of lockdowns, business and school closures, and quarantines, many individuals are home streaming more, and as such, they are using more of Netflix services.

Netflix stock price changed as follows:

March 11, 2020	stock price US$349.92
March 12, 2020	stock price US$315.25
March 16, 2020	stock price US$298.84
April 16, 2020	stock price US$439.17
April 23, 2020	stock price US$426.70

As you can see, had you bought Netflix at its lowest price on March 16, 2020, for US$298.84 and sold it at its highest price at US$439.17 on April 16, 2020, you would have made US$140.33 less fees. If you had bought one hundred (100) of these shares, you would have made US$14,033 less fees.

- Zoom

Zoom Video Communications Inc. is a communications technology company located in San Jose, California, U.S.A.

It trades on the NASDAQ with the symbol ZM.

Because of lockdowns, business and school closures, and quarantines, many individuals, employers, and employees, are teleconferencing, telecommunicating, doing their education and social relations via distance, so more of Zoom's services are being used.

Zoom stock price changed as follows:

March 11, 2020	stock price US$110.30
March 12, 2020	stock price US$109.47
March 13, 2020	stock price US$107.47
April 23, 2020	stock price US$169.09

As you can see, had you bought Zoom at its lowest price on March 13, 2020, for US$107.47 and sold it at its highest price at US$169.09 on April 23, 2020, you would have made US$61.62 less fees. If you had bought one hundred (100) of these shares, you would have made US$6,162 less fees.

- Facebook

Facebook Inc. is a social media technology company located in Menlo Park, California, U.S.A.

It trades on the NASDAQ with the symbol FB.

Because of lockdowns, business and school closures, and quarantines, many individuals, employers, and employees, are communicating and entertaining themselves via social media, so more of Facebook's services are being used.

Facebook stock price changed as follows:

March 11, 2020	stock price US$170.24
March 12, 2020	stock price US$154.47
March 16, 2020	stock price US$146.01
April 23, 2020	stock price US$185.13

As you can see, had you bought Facebook at its lowest price on March 16, 2020, for US$146.01 and sold it at its highest price at US$185.13 on April 23, 2020, you would have made US$39.12 less fees. If you had bought one hundred (100) of these shares, you would have made US$3,912 less fees.

- Shandong Dawn Polymer Co Ltd

Shandong Dawn Polymer Co Limited is a manufacturer that develops and sells polymer composite, and has dominated mask production in China.

These are the masks that China, and many other countries are purchasing to safeguard their health professionals, and citizens from the coronavirus.

It is located in Longkou, Shandong, China, and trades on the Shenzhen Stock Exchange (SHE) with the numbers 002838.

Shandong Dawn Polymer stock price (in Chinese Yuan) changed as follows:

January 2, 2020	stock price CNY$10.90
March 11, 2020	stock price CNY$51.20
March 12, 2020	stock price CNY$46.08
March 9, 2020	stock price CNY$59.00
April 23, 2020	stock price CNY$38.84

As you can see, had you bought Shandong Dawn Polymer on January 2, 2020, for CNY$10.90 (approx. US$1.54) and sold it at its highest price at CNY$59.00 (approx. US$8.33) on March 9, 2020, you would have made CNY$48.10 (approx. US$6.79) less fees. If you had bought one hundred (100) of these shares, you would have made US$679 less fees.

REAL ESTATE MARKET

As the pandemic continues, economies have slowed, and a recession is expected, a drop in housing prices are being anticipated. This is mainly because houses in markets such as in Canada and the U.S. are valued as overpriced.

For example, a house that is 1,794 sq. ft., 20-by-125 ft. lot, one car detached garage, 3 plus 1 bedroom, 4 bathrooms, two-storey detached, and finished basement was sold for CAD$1,700,000 on December 4, 2019, after it was bought for CAD$348,695 in 2008.

This house was located in the Avenue Rd. and Lawrence Ave. W. area in Toronto, Ontario, Canada.

PRECIOUS METALS

Precious metals like gold and silver are said to be great to maintain your wealth.

Gold prices have been on a steady increase, and have gone up even more since the pandemic.

Example of gold price movements are:

2018   gold price US$1,281.65

2019   gold price US $1,523.00

2020   gold price over US$1,726.50

Silver prices have been fluctuating, and have done more or less the same since the pandemic.

Example of silver price movements are:

2018   silver price US$15.52

2019   silver price US $17.90

2020   silver price approx. US$15.25

HEALTH

As stated in the introduction, a crisis is a time to reflect and deal with your mental, psychological, emotional, physical, and financial well-being.

Methods for improving and maintaining your overall health are:

1. Eat fruits and vegetables to get the nutrients you need.

ORGANIC FOOD & GROWING YOUR FOOD

Currently, there is a great demand for fresh farm food.

There is also demand for seeds to grow your food.

May I suggest getting a copy of the book *Why Organic Farming Is Great For Canada* (http://www.cariporterstore.biz/categories/organic-products-goods/organic-books-magazines-more.html), so you may learn more about organic goods, and growing your food.

It does not matter which country you live in; this book will be helpful.

2. Exercise regularly to help improve and maintain your health.

May I suggest the information below for inspiration, and to help you exercise at home wherever you are in the world.

Some of these entities do FREE zoom workouts as well.

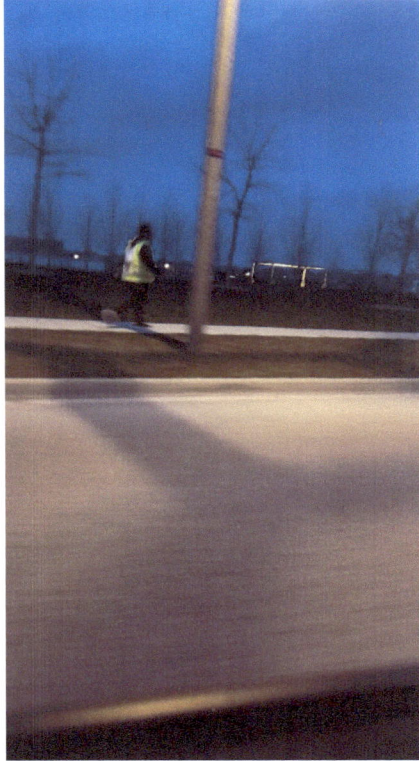

Even though the Run for Women event conducted by The LOVE YOU by Shoppers Drug Mart program in Canada was canceled due to the COVID-19 pandemic, Paula ran solo the 10K she had signed up for, and as part of her exercise routine.

Paula at HAZ2PEE YouTube Channel

https://www.youtube.com/channel/UCHpoqd-QcPD4h3C6yyiImLw

Urban Strength and Conditioning

https://urbanstrength.ca/

Abotti with Antonietta

https://abottiwithantonietta.ca/

3. Get sufficient sleep, so your body can recharge.

4. Keep yourself and surroundings clean, such as washing your hands and keeping surfaces hygienic.

Additional resources for helping to maintain and protect your mental health are:

CANADA

Canadian government website on protecting your mental health

https://www.canada.ca/en/public-health/services/protective-risk-factors-mental-health.html

Canadian government mental health services for kids and adults

https://www.canada.ca/en/public-health/services/mental-health-services.html

The U.S.

U.S. government mental help support and services

https://www.mentalhealth.gov/

Chapter Five – My War Against The Coronavirus COVID-19 Severe Acute Respiratory Syndrome Coronavirus 2 (SARS-COV-2)

The best defense against any illness is a robust immune system.

Your immune system is made up of biological parts and processes in your anatomy, and together they help to protect you from harmful substances, diseases, and organisms that may have entered into your body.

One way the immune system helps to protect you is by using phagocytes.

The phagocyte cells engulf things that enter the body, such as cells that cause gonorrhea, and kill them.

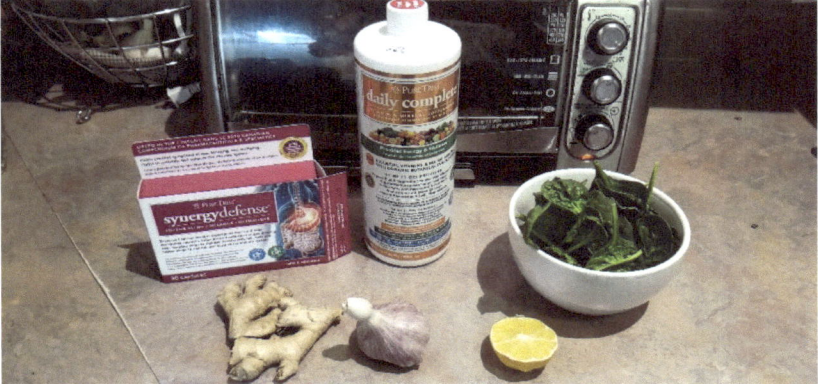

My Ammunition

Front L-R: ginger, garlic, lemon

Back L-R: Synergy Defense, Daily Complete, spinach

On a regular basis during winter, I use garlic and ginger as my flu shot. This natural way of preventing and recovering from the flu or cold has always worked for me, so it was a no brainer to continue during the SARS-COV-2 pandemic.

Because of how quickly SARS-COV-2 was spreading, so many individuals are dying, and as an essential worker on the frontlines, I decided to add more to my arsenal by using the supplements – Daily Complete and Synergy Defense.

It is just a little more; that way it is not overdone.

I eat my fruits like oranges and vegetables like spinach every day.

Daily, I will eat the ginger and garlic raw, or, I will consume them as tea with lemon and honey.

I always wash all fruits and vegetables with salt (has antibacterial properties), and water before consuming.

The supplements - Daily Complete, and Synergy Defense are taken on a regular basis to help maintain, and boost my immune system.

These supplements are available online worldwide at Cariporter Inc. Health Store (http://www.cariporterstore.biz/categories/organic-food-products-goods-others/cariporter-inc-health-store.html), where you can learn more as well.

GARLIC, GINGER, LEMON & HONEY TEA

When I decide to have the ginger and garlic as tea, I usually add lemon, and then honey to let it taste better.

The procedure is simple:

1. Boil the water

2. Peel and cut the ginger and garlic into small pieces

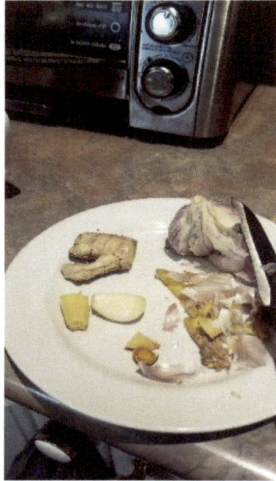

Ginger and garlic cut into small pieces

3. Cut a thin slice of lemon.

4. Place ginger, garlic, and lemon in your cup

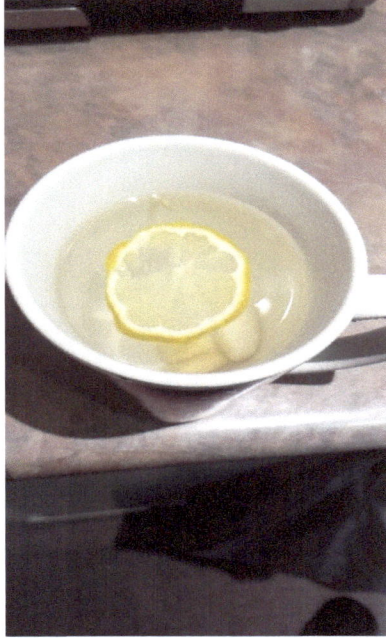

Ginger, garlic, and lemon in the cup with water

5. Place water in the cup.

   To increase potency, pour a small amount of
   water in the container just to cover the pieces and
   leave for about five (5) minutes.

Then pour the rest of hot water into the cup to your desired level.

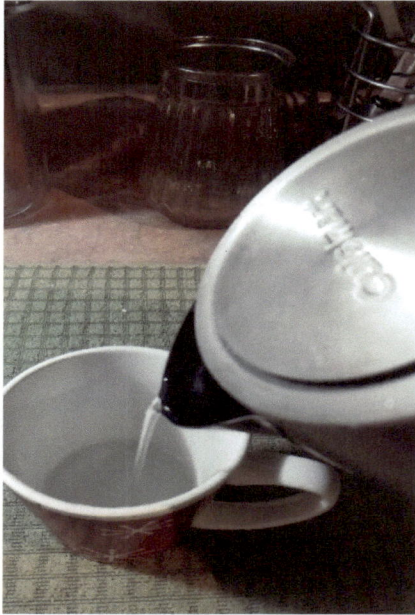

Pouring hot water into the cup

6. Mix tea with honey to taste.

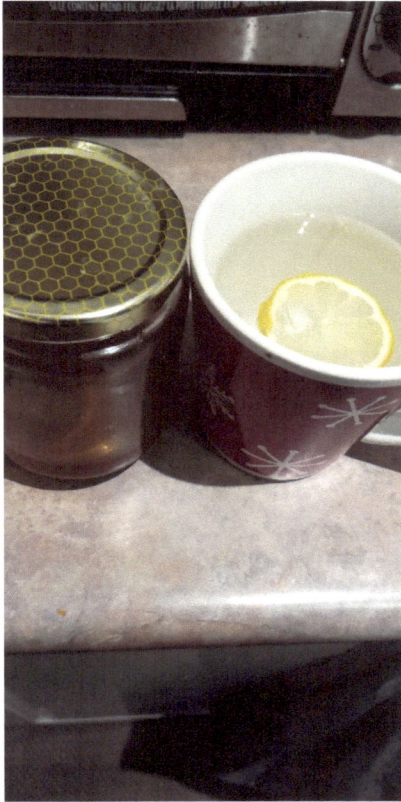

Honey jar beside cup

ABOUT THE AUTHOR

Leroy A. Brown is an organic farmer, author, speaker, and consultant.

Being an organic farmer, he has had to deal with adverse weather conditions and pests regularly. So it is normal for him to have to find ways of surviving economically.

Additionally, he became an organic farmer because of his interest in wanting to be healthy. And this interest he now shares with the world through his farm operation.

Therefore, it is no surprise that he has decided to share his knowledge, practices, and research globally, to help others navigate and become better from this current crisis.

You may follow him on:

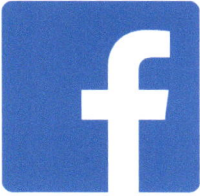

https://www.facebook.com/Leroy-A-Brown-1139168062882612/

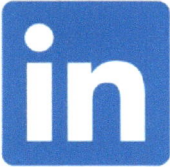

https://ca.linkedin.com/in/leroy-a-brown-268ba850

Other books written by Leroy A. Brown:

5. Why Organic Farming Is Great For Canada

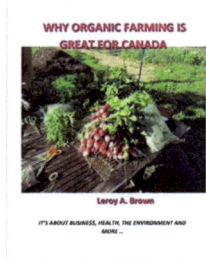

6. Natural Weight Loss, The Ultimate Guide With Easy To Do Recipes, Exercises And More … For Weight Loss

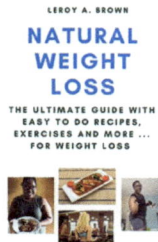

CONNECTING WITH CARIPORTER INC.

Cariporter Inc.

465 Yonge St. PO Box 73021,

Toronto, ON, M4Y 2W5, Canada

Tel: 1(647)852-4300

Email: info@cariporter.ca

Website: www.cariporter.ca

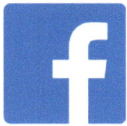

@ Cariporter Organic

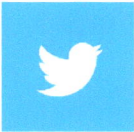

@ Cariporterstor1

@ Cariporter Inc

REFERENCES

<u>York Region Review</u> April 2020

<u>Financial Post</u> March 11, 2020

https://thecentsofmoney.com/eighteen-personal-finance-ratios-you-should-know/

https://www.economicshelp.org/blog/407/recession/who-benefits-from-a-recession/

https://www.incharge.org/financial-literacy/budgeting-saving/how-to-set-financial-goals/

https://www.iflscience.com/health-and-medicine/sarscov2-can-be-transmitted-via-shoes-and-spread-up-to-13-feet-in-the-air/

https://www.nerdwallet.com/blog/credit-cards/3-steps-spring-clean-card-debt/

https://www.mindtools.com/pages/article/smart-goals.htm

https://www.businessinsider.com/the-stock-market-crash-of-1929-what-you-need-to-know-2018-4

https://www.templeton.org/about/sir-john

INDEX

C

D

E

Emergency fund ratio 26

Emotional   12

Employment Insurance (EI)   74

Essential   10, 109

F

Federal Reserve   57, 58

Financial crisis 2007 – 2009   57

Financial security   10

Financial situation   11

G

Globe   11

Goals   13

Goods and Services Tax Credit   83

H

House 23

I

J

N

O

P

X

Y

Z

www.ingramcontent.com/pod-product-compliance
Lightning Source LLC
Chambersburg PA
CBHW040126270326
41927CB00001B/3